SimpleGuy Diet

www.simpleguydiet.com

SimpleGuy Diet

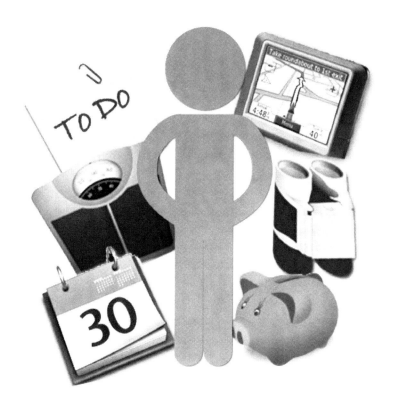

Skip Lei

Copyright © 2010 by Skip Lei. All rights reserved.
ISBN 978-1-105-27105-2

Dedication

This simple book is dedicated to **you**. Congratulations on taking the first step towards better health and lower weight by reading this book.

Meet the Simple Guy

I am a pathetically average 50-something male. I have a job, a wife, two kids, a house and a small yard to mow. I weighed just under 180 pounds when I graduated college and, over time, I slowly worked my way up to 212. That works out to about a pound a year of gain. I have always been healthy and have no medical issues, again, just pathetically normal.

My wife is smarter, more disciplined and a better athlete than me. Last year, on her birthday, she decided to start a slight lifestyle change to lose a bit of weight.

She forked over a small recurring monthly fee for some famous Internet diet program and immediately started to assign "points" to everything she consumed. She joined an online group and rallied some of her friends to start walking with her every day. This sounded crappy to me; everything she was doing sounded like work, and thus, I had no interest in mirroring her strategy.

In my small-minded way, I decided to focus on a couple super-simple food adjustments just to see what would happen. With virtually no effort in my first three months, I lost seven pounds. The next month I lost four more pounds and then three additional pounds fell off. No pills, no counting points, no gym membership, no equipment to buy—just simple self-managed changes.

Now, after six months, I have taken about 20 pounds off of my starting weight and I'm in love with this low-effort process!

Many of my friends and co-workers ask me how this happened. They invite me to lunch or for a cup of coffee to have a little "one on one time" to extract the magic of my weight loss. What I have decided to do is spend some time to have a website created and populate it with simple information to better share my success. After thousands of visits to our website (www.simpleguydiet.com), I was urged to publish this booklet and have The Simple Guy Diet available to those who would prefer a paperback rather than a download. I have worked hard to keep the publishing/distribution costs as low as possible to deliver the best possible value for your hard-earned money. Please enjoy the information and the adventure of this simple weight loss story.

I know this is what worked for me..... and, hopefully, it will work for you too!

My Inspiration

People often ask my why I created the Simple Guy Diet. It was part out of personal need, part sharing my success, part creating accessibility to friends and family and part based on inspiration from a couple of business books I read years ago.

Have you ever read the books FISH! (Stephen Lundin) or The One Minute Manager (Ken Blanchard)? They are wonderfully short, yet profoundly affecting business related books; one is about organizational development and the other is about general leadership. Neither will make you a specialist on either topic, but what each will do is share a story or two for you to adapt into your own world. Rather than "how-to," The One Minute Manager and FISH! focus on business situations that will hopefully inspire you to think differently and potentially find new solutions which lead to change. On a personal level, the style of each of these books really clicked for me…and I believe, to the millions of others who read them.

The "voice" and message of The Simple Guy Diet is somewhat the same. The Simple Guy Diet is a story of a real person, me, and my simplified approach to lowering the number on my bathroom scale. This is *not* a step by step "how to" diet book chock-a-block full of recipes, but rather, a "one guy to another" story respecting both your precious time and hard earned money.

Simple Guy Diet

Please enjoy this quick read and apply it to your own life and unique set of circumstances. With a small and focused commitment, you will be happily taking your first step to a healthier you!!

My To-Do List

1. Commit to 30 days
2. Buy a digital scale
3. Have a food road map
4. Celebrate your inner-cheapness
5. Enjoy the view

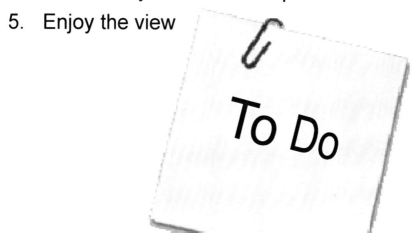

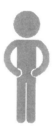

Commit to 30 Days

Commit to 30 Days

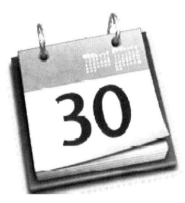

Before you do anything, you need to select an official day to start and declare it as law!

To give yourself the best chance at success, try to start where you have no big "eating" events in the first couple of weeks like the Super Bowl, an office party or your neighborhood block party. I found it best to start on a Sunday so you can control what you do the day before falling into your soon to change workweek routine.

Remember, you are *not* changing forever, just for 30 days to see if this adjustment fits your lifestyle. Once you get to your 30-day anniversary, then, if you have been successful, it is your choice to continue. I started with 30 days and have not stopped. In fact, it just gets easier and more empowering!

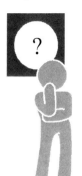

So, are you in for 30 days?

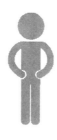

Buy a Digital Scale

Buy a Digital Scale

Rather than spending money on pills, special foods or online programs, I strongly suggest you go to your local store, department store, on-line retailer, Walmart or Target and buy a DIGITAL scale.

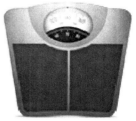

You really need to have a scale before your first day. This will start you on the road to honesty. My wife is a big believer in the scale and hops on it every morning. For the first month, I weighed myself every Monday morning before I took my shower. It is important that you find a time to serve as your "baseline weigh-in time". Your weight naturally fluctuates during the course of the day, so pick a time that works best for you and weigh-in the same time and same day of the week for your first four weeks. After your first month, I would recommend that you weigh yourself every day (at the same time each day).

The great part of a digital scale is that it is brutally accurate. After my initial month of weight loss, which was seven pounds for me, I started to focus on the last two digits of the scale for my morning, pre-shower, weigh in. As an example:

If the scale read 196.4, I would tell myself "64," representing the last two digits.

The next day I might be "62" and in several days "54." I found this to be both rewarding and motivating by just focusing on the last two numbers. This way, every little change, even a tenth of a pound, felt like a personal victory—and a great reason to stick to the plan.

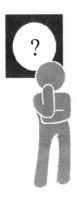 Are you willing to get a digital scale?

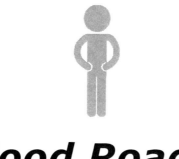

My Food Road Map

My Food Road Map

I refuse to have things be difficult, I chose a logical and unscientific approach..... as I am both logical and unscientific.

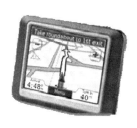

I eliminated "obvious" carbs from my diet. From my very first day, I gave up all bread, rice, potatoes and tortillas (and I love tortillas!). I certainly was NOT carb free. I continued to eat my bowl of instant oatmeal with a handful of Post grape-nuts, a palm full of crushed walnuts and a quarterish-cup of 1% milk as I had always had for breakfast. I also eliminated most desserts for the first month. When I need a sweet fix, I do occasionally have a cut up apple sprinkled with cinnamon and sugar or a coffee mug full of regular vanilla yogurt and grape-nuts as my evening dessert.

SOME RANDOM TIPS:

- If it is white, don't eat it (bread, rice, potatoes, tortillas, etc.)
- Eliminate most soft drinks and replace with water (I added a pinch of Crystal Light lemonade powder for a little flavor, but just a pinch)

- Adios to french fries, adios to onion rings and adios to anything that is cooked in a fryer
- Keep a pack of gum in your car or any other place you typically want to snack. Sometimes keeping your mouth occupied with gum can prevent unneeded snacking
- Find things that are not bad for you to fall in love with (for me it was a tall americano at Starbucks)
- Just say no to desserts, doughnuts (I love doughnuts even more than I do tortillas) and anything in a bakery case

THINGS THAT HAPPENED TO ME:

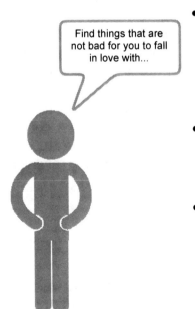

Find things that are not bad for you to fall in love with...

- I craved crunchy!! I loved having a half dozen baby carrots or a handful of raw almonds for a snack; almonds are great for the office too
- For some weird reason, I had a coffee mug full of red wine most evenings, but just one
- For the first time in my life, I ate dark chocolate (at least 70% cocoa); I would have a piece the size of two to four postage stamps (also, keep it in the fridge, it's a million times better)

LUNCH IDEAS:

Since I work for a pretty big company, many times I do not have the time for a full hour to eat. Coupled with the fact that packing my own lunch was not a good option (too un-fun) for me the following worked:

1. Go to McDonalds and order a side salad and a McDouble (each off the dollar menu) and a cup of water. Use no more than 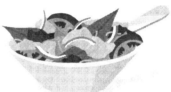 25% of the dressing packet, put the lid back on and shake it up. As for the McDouble, take the top and the bottom bun off and move it aside. With what is left, take the plastic knife from the salad kit and cut the burger into multiple pieces, making it last a bit longer. I hate to admit this, but I went to McDonalds two or three times a week, so I had to find how to make this habit fit into a diet regimen. Try to modify some of your favorites, so you aren't feeling too restricted in your new lifestyle.

2. If you happen to have a Costco or grocery store nearby, purchase the pre-made chicken Caesar salad. Do not put on the croutons and use no more than half of the salad dressing offered. Again, place the lid back on, and while holding the lid, shake it like crazy to get it all mixed up. Eat half and save the other half for your lunch the next day. Be sure to keep the plastic fork in the container, as finding a replacement fork the next day can be problematic. Hopefully you have a fridge at work to store your food treasure for the next day.

3. If you are a "brown-bagger", be sure that two things happen: 1) Keep it as carb-free as possible and 2) Pack things you like and look forward to consuming. This will allow you to become the master of your own happiness!

DINNER IDEAS:

1. Personally, I have had *great* success with buying bags of salad at my local grocery store. Do *not* buy the ones with dressing in the bag, as many times these are packaged with other evil things....like won-ton sticks in the oriental salad. Add different veggies you may have on hand to maintain variety and that all important CRUNCH. I use a squirt of Hidden Valley Ranch Dressing and a generous amount of black pepper. Most weeks I buy a pre-cooked baked rotisserie chicken at the grocery store and cut up a piece to mix in with my salad.

2. I try to find some kind of meat or fish as my main entree (rather than a monster salad as my main dish) once or twice a week. When I do, my evening glass of red wine seems to get consumed for dinner (again, you only get one!). Add a side of steamed veggies or a small salad and you're good to go! I learned (from my wife) to really slow down and stretch out the time it takes to consume the meal, excellent advice indeed! If buying a pre-made chicken or barbecuing meat isn't happening, then a lightly doctored up can of tuna will also do the trick.

3. Bad news, my brothers, steer clear of beer.

DON'T FORGET DESSERT:

- A cut up apple sprinkled with cinnamon and sugar
- A small piece of dark chocolate
- A small coffee mug (portion) of wine...assuming you are of legal drinking age!
- A small coffee mug with yogurt and grape-nuts

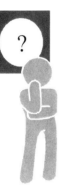

What simple changes will you be making?

The Simple Guy's Dining Out Favorites

Old Problem		New Solution
Burger		Lose the bun, lose the mayo and wrap that burger in lettuce. My local McDonald's, In-N-Out, Burger King and Five Guys are all happy to sell you the burger of your choice without the bun
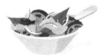 Salad		Ditch the croutons and ask for the dressing on the side (using no more than half of the dressing!) I also take the first bite before adding the dressing
Omelette		An excellent choice is an omelette, but get it al a carte, without the toast or the hash browns. This will be good for ANY meal of the day....in any country

Have fun creating your own new solutions!

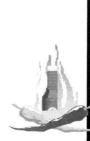

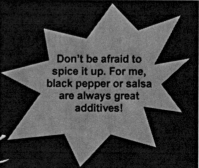

Don't be afraid to spice it up. For me, black pepper or salsa are always great additives!

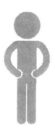

Be the Genius Salad Maker You Know You Are

Be the Genius Salad Maker You Know You Are

Nobody knows what you like more than you!! Now, the goal is how to create the ultimate win-win food; a salad that is "look-forward-to-good" and still allows you to work toward your weight reduction goal. Below are some good things to 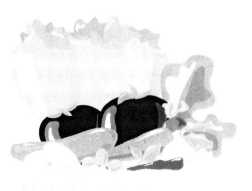 think about before you dive in. Hopefully, these tips will get you started on your pathway to salad preparation success.

SALAD MAKING TIPS:

- Clean out your fridge of foods you no longer need as these are distractions
- Purchase two or three of your favorite dressings (I have two)
- Dedicate yourself to become the best salad maker you know
- Find ways to treat yourself with salad "additives"

Simple Guy Diet

- Don't be afraid to add things that you never had in a salad before
- Find a "master bowl" to call your own…and use the same one each night for dinner (for me, I have a bowl that is capable of holding six cups of water. My salads only fills about half the bowl, the extra room makes it ideal to mix up without creating a major mess)
- Use a different beverage on different nights to help add variety to your daily masterpiece
- Purchasing bags of lettuce in your local grocery store is a great way to simplify and find plenty of variety with your cornerstone ingredient
- Rule the vegetable aisle; be sure to have plenty of other veggies on hand to mix in, and when you know things are not healthy add-ins, play fair

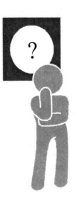

What is your favorite masterpiece salad?

THE 60-30-10 PLAN:

I have found this to be a good working proportion in my salad making creations. I have 60% of my bowl contents be lettuce + (lettuce from a head or from a store bought bag), 30% will be what I call "healthy additives" and 10% "bad stuff". Below is an expanded explanation to give you a better idea of each ingredient category:

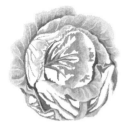

Lettuce + (60%)

- Pre-packaged (about 1/3 of a bag equals one serving)
- Whole head (about 1/4 head equals one serving)
- Shredded slaw to mix in

Healthy Additives (30%)

- A palm full of shelled sunflower seeds
- A palm full of chopped nuts
- Baby carrots
- Freshly chopped veggies
- Grilled veggies
- Spiced up tofu
- Lean meat or fish of your choice (4 ounces)
- Ground pepper
- Avocado
- Chopped fresh fruit
- Salsa

Bad Stuff (10%)

- Salad Dressing (one heaping tablespoon)
- Ice cream scoop size of tuna or chicken salad
- Palm full of crunched up Ruffles potato chips (really!)
- Croutons (palm full)
- Tablespoon of BBQ sauce
- A palm full of shredded cheese

One of the questions I receive is, "What is your favorite masterpiece salad?" About once a week I really go for it and make what I believe to be is my ultimate salad, which I affectionately refer to as my "Heaven and Hell Salad." Although the ingredients vary from week to week, it may contain the following:

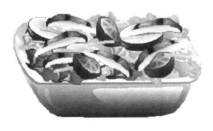

- ½ of a medium sized avocado
- 6 BBQ Ruffle potato chips, crushed up
- One heaping tablespoon of ranch dressing
- 1/3 bag of store bought heart of romaine lettuce (in my "master bowl")
- A palm full of shelled sunflower seeds
- Two tablespoons of medium ground pepper (that's a ton…but I love it!)
- A palm full of cut up chicken
- 1/3 of a cucumber, diced
- 6 baby carrots
- 6 baby tomatoes cut in half

I realize my masterpiece may not be for everyone, but certainly you will identify your own dinner work of art. Remember, to keep variety in what you make. If you are anything like me, you will have a couple of "go to" salads which always do the trick. At first, the building and the creation part is what I liked least...but now, it is absolutely my favorite part and I feel I am the king of the veggie aisle at my local grocery store......and, it's good to be king!

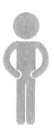

Celebrate Your Inner Cheapness

Celebrate Your Inner Cheapness

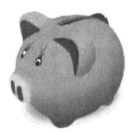

For me, the joy of spending less money was almost as fun as watching the pounds melt away.

Not purchasing bread items, desserts, beer, chips and processed snacks clearly was a money saver. Discovering low carb ways to eat off the dollar menu and living without soda was a huge eye opener. Things like baby carrots and buying a pre-packaged whole cooked chicken at the local grocery store will highlight what great values there are when you eat in a sensible, low-carb way.

If you and your family are going out to eat, have a small self-managed snack (either 10 baby carrots, or a banana, or handful of almonds) while you are waiting for your team to saddle up before you go out. Then, at the restaurant, drink only water (or iced tea or coffee if you want to go a bit crazy financially) and have the house salad. In the words of my Italian friend, Guido, "No bread!" This is the key to the kingdom....and a most evil table temptation!

What you will quickly see, as I have, is how much you spend when you eat out for things that aren't at all beneficial to you. Eating consciously, more fresh and in a low-carb manner will save you a ton of money!

Also, a good food source for those daily lunches or simple take home evening meals, is in a full service grocery store with a deli counter. Most of the larger regional and national grocery chain stores offer various premade options. As an example, for a lunch, I would set a budget of $4. Then I would choose from the deli counter, eliminating anything that has been fried. No orange chicken, no egg rolls, no corn dogs and avoid anything with big carbs like potato salad and pasta salad. Be sure one of the items is veggie-based. I have found this to be a great way to get a big and adventurous bang for my buck and it is an awesome trick for dinners as well!

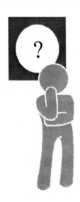

What can you think of to change it up?

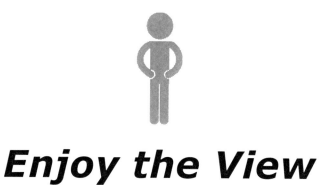

Enjoy the View

Enjoy the View

I was an athlete in high school and athletic in college. Sports had always been an important part of my life.

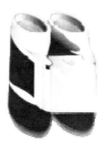

Sometime in my mid-40s, the weekly basketball pick-up games stopped, I lost all interest in running in organized events, my gym membership (which I still have) has become little more than a recurring monthly bill and no longer did I have much interest in playing tennis.

I still very much love all of these activities, but rarely do them.....and if/when I do, it is not with any regularity. Somehow, I am now more concerned about avoiding injury than I am about being physically active or competitive. It sounds weird, but it is true.

My wife, as I mentioned earlier, started walking....big time. On the weekends she would walk me like a dog!! At first I scoffed at this, as it is *not* a sport and it certainly is *not* athletic. I have now grown to love our long, cruising around weekend walks—no matter what the weather. There is no equipment necessary (other than your favorite pair of Nikes) or team to join. Best of all, excuses not to do it are out the window! Fitness aside, I have also found this a great time to get caught up on last week's events, as well as get clear on what's cooking for next week with my wife or, if you go it alone, a super time to work through issues or just to think creatively. On many levels, walking has been a huge game changer for me both physically and emotionally!

I can't believe I'm saying this, but walking is cool. By hoofing it around I am seeing my local world in a whole new way..... and just enjoying the view.

SYNERGIZE YOUR NEEDS (MULTI-TASK!)
1. Listen to a book on MP3 while walking
2. Make yard work part of your scheduled workout
3. Assign yourself physical chores
4. Do some physical activities with the kids
5. Think long and hard about the day/week ahead while walking
6. Wash your car by hand, just like your dad did
7. The stairs are your friend, visit them often
8. Walk a mile or two to your favorite coffee place
9. Mentally align yourself for a great week at work
10. Psychoanalyze your friends and family members

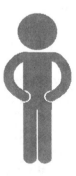

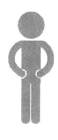

We All Stumble....

We All Stumble....

Worry not, Simple Guys, as we all stumble a bit from time to time, it's a "guy thing!"

Although you will be enjoying the fruits of your success as the pounds fall off with your new eating game plan, you will have small bursts of time when your weight is going the wrong way.

The good news (about the bad news) is that you will know why your scale is creeping northbound. There has likely been a "situation / event" which has taken you off your Simple Guy game. It just happens. The school reunion, a wedding weekend packed with activities, a family vacation, an extended birthday / anniversary celebration or a multi-day off-site meeting / conference for work are, for me, just plain bad.

I have found that a multi-hour one-day event like a neighborhood block party, a football game watch party or an evening out with friends is totally manageable and only a little "slippage" may occur. But once I get into the multi-day events, I really seem to fall back to my ways of old, even when I think I am managing them! Snacks, treats, chips and salsa seem to not only appear, but be calling my name. Even though I am conscious of what I am eating (which may be a victory by itself), I still onboard much more than I would when I am controlling my own routine.

I have learned that when I am out of my "controlled environment", I eat differently and ultimately gain a few pounds—to which I say, "Big deal!" The silver lining is that I now know that once I get back into my successful Simple Guy routine, in about a week (not a day or two), I will be back to my pre-vacation weight and right on track to slowly and sensibly lose more.

Keep the faith, my brothers, and happily know that the bumps in the road can be easily smoothed out.

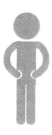

I Changed More Than My Weight

I Changed More Than My Weight

It's official.....at least in my mind..... that change has indeed occurred! Certainly I have dropped at least one jeans/pant size and my weight loss is now seemingly visible to all who know me. Here are several call outs of BIG things, which happened as the result of dropping some pounds over the first six months:

1. I am not as interested in impulse food consumption as I was in the past.
2. I am making better food choices and it seems absolutely natural to me.
3. I am shocked when I watch others eat (by choice and quantity) and can't believe that was once me!
4. I gave away a bunch of jeans and pants to Goodwill. Before this experience, I was always too cheap to give them away as I might need them again.
5. I feel as if I am not compromising with my food intake; rather, I'm just living in a new and better way.
6. I learned that losing weight, for me, was not about the food or the number on a scale. It was more about understanding my "triggers," like celebrating my inner-cheapness, keeping it simple and *NOT* being told what to do that made this work for me.

7. I love doughnuts! Although I did not have a doughnut for the first couple of months, when I did have one, it was absolutely awesome! Treating yourself every now and then is not a crime.
8. I am thrilled with being a "junior walk-a-holic," as somehow in the past couple of years, physical activity got put on the back burner. Even though I am not working up a great sweat by walking, I love every step I take.
9. I now know that I could indeed lose even more weight by increasing my exercise habits or adjusting my food once again. At this point I am pretty darn happy where I am and, after six months, I am down about 20 pounds and still creeping down bit by bit.

Please remember, this is not a prescription or a guarantee. It is just something that worked very well for me. It is always a good idea to check in with your doctor before doing anything different. I wish you all the success in the world. Please have fun doing this for 30 days (and play fair) and see where it leads you. Everyone is different and being successful needs to be absolutely unique to you.

Do it for yourself......change is good!!!

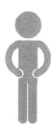

Simple Guy BLOG Wisdom

Simple Guy BLOG Wisdom

As time marches on, so do the posts on the Simple Guy website. I thought it would be good to share some of the thoughts and emotions I had while in my first six months of weight loss, as well as my thinking and observations in the months that followed.......

GENERAL BLOG POSTS:

+ *I am still surprised on the rare occasion when I look in the mirror.....not only by my loss of weight, but also that I have been successful in doing so*

+ *My Starbucks americanos are still very important to me....so much so, that when I am in a restaurant or at home, I am having hot tea which makes my Starbucks run even more special*

+ *I am having a blast using the "wrong dishes" when I eat. Many times I will use coffee mug at home rather than a bowl....or in a self service place or a place where we are served "family style", I am using a saucer or a coffee cup to replace a full size plate or a bowl*

+ *Missing meals or not eating my usual things seem to get me slightly off track. I find the greatest success to starting my day off with a very small bowl of oatmeal and then just stick to MY plan has been the best strategy (for me)*

+ My love for cold cereal (and was my "go to option" for a fast dinner) is totally gone. With the exception of a shot of Grape Nuts in my morning oatmeal....or in some yogurt at night

+ Now that I am down around 20 pounds, I also think that my posture is better. I am not sure that it actually is, but I seem more conscious of being more "upright"

+ Finish strong!! One thing that I have learned is when I do eat out, make my last bite a great one. I reserve some of the best things from my order to have my last bite be my best

+ Own it!! Once you lose your first 5 pounds....you need to feel like you "own" that weight and are not going back. You should be at that weight or lower for a week to have full ownership; then focus to lose the next five....once there, own that number. Hitting a "target weight" is good....but without "owning it", it will just be a moment in time

+ Before the SG, going to bed was the most anticipated part of my day; but now, bedding down is a bit of a downer as I can not wait to get rollin' the next morning

+ According to my wife and kids, I rarely snore....which certainly WAS NOT the case before my weight loss

+ I have the opportunity to work with some awesome people. One gal, about my age has boundless energy and focus. Not sure how she does it, but I bet part of it is that she eats right , as my energy and my ability to "fire up" in the morning has been a noticeable and dramatic change

+ This is kooky....now I have happily fallen into a rhythm of food consistency/regularity (oatmeal for breakfast and a medium salad bar serving for lunch). I find myself only wanting the same things for each meal. Before I met the SG, I was fueled and energized by variety (Baskin Robbins, Noah's bagels, TGI Fridays....), but now places like this feel somewhere between distracting and overwhelming. I am really liking my simplistic, repetitive pattern.....as it too, has made my life less fussy

+ For some reason I have started to try and do a bit of "ab work". I have this goofy roller-thing that my wife bought on an infomercial (OK, maybe I bought it, but it was years ago)...so now I do just 12 in the morning and 12 in the evening (the first time I did 25 I was crazy-sore for 3 days!). Not sure if it will do anything...but at least it will satisfy my urge to "try"....

+ My "enough" is now noticeably less than when I started the SG lifestyle. Smaller portions are what I crave....big portions of anything seem to live somewhere between "wrong and just plain bad"

+ As my portions have become smaller, I find myself gravitating to smaller pates and bowls to put my food on. My full-sized bowls and plates in my kitchen now rarely used (by me)

+ Somehow my new beverage of choice is a cup of water with no ice and just a splash of 7-Up. It may sound weird, but for me, it is way better than just water.....and way better for me than a soft drink

+ I have never been a big salad guy till I started rollin' with the Simple Guy. Before quantity was a requirement of each meal .....but now, being super selective at a salad bar and making a small (or at least smaller) masterpiece is really working well for me

+ I seem to have lost interest in fast food burgers....rarely going there anymore....except with my teenage son. I wonder (when I was hooked on McDonald's for the first 3-4 months) if this was just a natural need to stay connected to my eating past....the food...the ordering process....the tray....the surroundings....it is certainly a mystery to me

+ My weight has stabilized.... even with more regular indulgences

+ Portioned and infrequent indulgences: 1 (not 2 or 3 like before) donuts every couple of weeks......a small piece of bread to dip into olive oil at an Italian restaurant

+ Fork fulls to win!..... I have found that a fork is a pretty darn handy way to indulge. It serves as an excellent "portion control devise". If I decide to have a little piece of brownie.....before grabbing a square, I now use a fork and my only decision is if I'm going to have one or two fork fulls....eat it, love it and walk away

+ Most of us have heard the term, "cheat to win"....but for the Simple Guy, I have now adopted the philosophy of "Swipe to Win." By successfully swiping (with permission, of course) a couple of bites of my wife's sweet potatoes or a fork full of her dessert....this gives me a wonderfully satisfying taste of my past without being confronted with entire portion to (likely mis-) manage myself

+ A better fast food option for me (at this moment) is Taco Bell (for me, it's not about the food there....it's their darn hot sauce that I crave). One "fresco taco" with hot sauce is so sinfully good. Never be fooled....tortillas are evil....even the little ones!! Make this a weekly treat at most

+ Still nothing seems worth having in the Starbucks treat case....although I still go to Starbucks about 10 times a week for my tall americano. There have been times when I purchased a single banana....I always wondered who bought bananas there.....

+ I was rollin' for a while by having the barista add foam to my americano (a tall foamy americano if you want to try one). That was great for a couple of months, but I have now bounced back to one without foam

+ My daily ritual of high cocoa content chocolate has mysteriously ended. I am not sure what the insight is here, but it is clear that some cravings have "just ended"

+ Ready for my next run to Goodwill. I have a pile of clothes (now shirts are included) that were "on the bubble" with regard to fit and size.....now, I have no interest in keeping them

+ Still no running for the Simple Guy, but my tennis racquet is re- strung and I have had several (very fun) "social hits" a couple times a month

+ Oatmeal = control!! I now find myself taking my (stupid) instant oatmeal packets, a plastic spoon and crushed walnuts when I travel for personal reasons. I do love oatmeal...but I also feel it gives me both control and a sense of protection from being victimized by whatever there might (and might not) be available for breakfast

+ I am really into drinking warm water in the morning and hot water with many of my meals

+ Holy smokes....I just went through the TSA line in the airport. When the agent handed me back my license, I noticed that my weight was lower than stated....for the first time in 20 years I won't need to "round down" my weight when I renew my license!

+ People seem to always ask me if I have more energy since I lost the weight. In general, I would say no.....although maybe I do, but since the change was so darn gradual, I just have not been able to tell

+ This is weird, but I seem to wake up an hour earlier (new for me) AND at full speed (REALLY NEW for me). This is indeed a change....and I must say, one of the best outcomes of my weight loss!!

+ I am still living in the halo of accolades about my visible weight loss. I wish I had something more magical to tell them.....but really, for me, it is nothing more than hangin' with the Simple Guy

+ Beer has fallen off my radar....really not sure why....but my interest is near zero

+ Things that were indulgences before (a big milk shake, a vanilla bean frappiccino, a peanut buster parfait at Dairy Queen) seem to be nearly impossible consumption items now. I am not trying not to want them.....they just don't hold the same "temptation value" as in the past

+ I am becoming a bit of a "label-looker". In the past, I rarely looked at the nutrition facts; as frankly, I was just not interested. I still am not. However, now I do give it the occasional glance to how it rates with carbohydrates. When you're not sure about what you might be ready to consume, a quick look is a pretty darn good thing to do. I ended up with a little...and I mean little box of raisins and thought, "This MUST be a healthy choice....they're raisins". Once I checked the facts, I realized that little box had 10% of my daily carb value! I took a pass, but in the past would have happily consumed the box in a bite or two

+ When dining out, do yourself a favor and have your menu item selected before you sit down. It is just too darn easy to have the chicken Caesar salad (you thought you were going to order) turn into mozzarella sticks and a personal pan pizza once staring at the menu!!

+ When you go out and order a salad, remember these 5 words of wisdom, "Dressing on the side, please!".....it will be a game changer and keep YOU in total control

+ I used to not be satisfied till I was full....and I mean physically full....no room left. Now, on the rare occasion that I am stuffed, if feels both bad and just "wrong"

SIMPLE GUY STORIES:

+ I am a bit bummed out by the food consumption of others. I am certainly not a judgmental person, but I kind of feel that way when watching others eat. In a recent flight for work to Europe I sat next to 3 sisters (ages 60-70) flying over the Atlantic on vacation. My usual gig is to eat something I choose to eat at the airport and pass on the first meal on the plane. Within an hour of take-off, a monster egg-salad sandwich and a big bag of Kettle Chips emerged from one of their carry-ons. They were like three wild dogs sharing their prey as they passed this monstrous mess back and forth to each other. Within the 90 minutes, our airplane meal came....I passed.....and they consumed!! A round of raviolis, a dinner roll, cheese and crackers, a small salad with dressing and a brownie were licked clean. Gold stars for them!! Hours later I woke up from my nap and the food-sisters we knocking down a giant piece of chocolate cake they had carried on as well....this chocolate beast was about the same volume as a half a carton of cigarettes. Not a crumb survived. Our pre-landing omelet was met with the same enthusiasm......where does all the food go?....and man, am I THRILLED that I am not like that anymore!

+ Your weight is like flying a jet. I took a week off of work to have a little bonus family time. While off that week, it seems I had totally lost control of what food I was confronted with.....and ultimately consuming! The days seemed to be focused around "favorite places to eat"....not to mention hanging with friends and family which too, made "eating right" tough for me. After the first several days of "bad behavior", my weight had not really changed.....foolishly, I believed that my new life style had perhaps created the antidote for the consumption of guacamole and chips, pizza and peanut M & Ms. Near the end of my week-o-fun, my weight was hopping up about a pound a day. The following work week I reverted back to my Simple Guy way of living. Equally foolish, I thought a day or two would do the trick....in reality it took another 5-8 days to get back and "own" my desired weight. The moral to the story is.....you can't blow OR fix your weight in a single day....or two. The best analogy I can think of is that our weight is like flying a jet plane. It takes a while to get the plane rolling with enough speed to achieve lift-off......conversely, it takes a long time to slow a jet plane down. Any change, good or bad, will require you to have a longer (than you might think) runway of time to see results.

VACATION POSTS:

+ On our annual week-long vacation/family reunion, the chips, cookies and assorted kid-friendly boxed-snacks never got consumed....at least by me. Although a couple of red vines did find their way into my possession

+ *I am still craving my daily oatmeal and grape nuts every morning. In fact I brought the stuff with me on the family get away...it was both comforting and helped me steer clear from the daily homemade scones and sticky buns*

+ *On vacation I had a blast playing golf several times....but also walking 6-10 miles (by choice) everyday.....in fact, I couldn't get enough (OK, the weather was awesome)!! I am now an official "walkaholic"....not one of those goofy super fast guys or the dude carrying weights, but rather just walking "with a purpose".....about 18 minute miles.....or 3.5 miles per hour*

+ *When traveling near or far, consider an omelet....pass on the toast and the potatoes....as a good "travel anytime meal" alternative*

Be sure to check in from time to time on the Simple Guy BLOG ..... Simply by logging on to our website at: **www.simpleguydiet.com**

About the author

Skip Lei is a self-proclaimed pathetically average 50-something male with a job, a wife, two kids and a small yard to mow. Happily living in the Pacific Northwest, he gave up on weight loss and blamed an unfairly slow metabolism and a lack of commitment for his creeping weight.

Realizing that most diet programs were too structured or too alien, he simply created his own life-style fitting method to see what would happen. He would be the first to admit that his weight loss story is not cosmic.....he would also smile knowing he shed nearly 10% of his body weight and is no longer referred to as a "chubby-hubby".

NOTES

The reason we needed to have these final

NOTES

blank pages is to meet a requirement in

NOTES

publishing. I had the option to add

NOTES

additional content but refused; as the whole

NOTES

purpose of this book was to be simple and

NOTES

concise. Please use these "bonus" pages to

NOTES

write/capture meaningful notes, or just rip

NOTES

them out, cut them into little pieces and use

NOTES

as scrap paper to create grocery lists for

NOTES

the next four weeks. Enjoy!

Lightning Source UK Ltd.
Milton Keynes UK
UKOW05f1251151213

223034UK00002B/13/P